Mema's Ramblings
on being well

Mema's Ramblings
on being well

✦

a guide so that everyone can be well and have ultimate wellness at age 75

Freddie Martin Arbuthnot

iUniverse, Inc.

New York   Bloomington

Mema's Ramblings on being well
a guide so that everyone can be well and have ultimate wellness at age 75

iUniverse books may be ordered through booksellers or by contacting:

iUniverse
1663 Liberty Drive
Bloomington, IN 47403
www.iuniverse.com
1-800-Authors (1-800-288-4677)

Because of the dynamic nature of the Internet, any Web addresses or links contained in this book may have changed since publication and may no longer be valid. The views expressed in this work are solely those of the author and do not necessarily reflect the views of the publisher, and the publisher hereby disclaims any responsibility for them.

ISBN: 978-1-4502-1403-2 (sc)
ISBN: 978-1-4502-1404-9 (ebk)

Printed in the United States of America

iUniverse rev. date: 2/15/2010

Chapter One

Introduction

The subtitle of this little book could be: How to be 75 years old and have optimal wellness. It does not matter if your life is in a downward spiral or on auto pilot just breezing along, you can create lifetime wellness by changing your focus on lifestyle and taking charge of your attitude and health. The sky is your limit. You can't manage the world but you can manage your life with your decisions. I made a decision to stay well several years ago and even though I stray from my wellness program from time to time, I soon get back on the road to "staying well". As I see people who have chronic illness, it makes me more determined than ever to live my life in ultimate wellness. I was told by a family member that the reason I did not get sick was because, I am stubborn competitive and determined to always win. I don't know if that was supposed to be a compliment or not, I think not.

I have made this little book easy to read and short so that you will have fun reading it and will finish it. As you read this it will not take you long to realize that I am not at all pleased with the present day medical system.

You can take as long as you want implementing your own wellness program but read all my ramblings before you begin implementing your wellness program.

When I was working as a registered nurse in the traditional medical world, I often questioned the health care provider about providing wellness for the patient and they usually completely ignored me, I think that was because they did not know how to keep people well but always treated their illnesses one after the other. You would think that all those patients with high blood pressure would have an order to eat several stalks of celery a day, or the heart patient be required to have fresh pineapple every day, these ideas are just randomly chosen but it is a shame that the health care provider is not educated about the natural healing of foods and supplements.

I started studying about wellness and the holistic approach to treatment of illness, as a young mother. After many years of frustration and stress until I retired from nursing in the traditional world of medicine, I kept studying. At that time information was limited and was usually considered "folk medicine". Much of my knowledge now can be traced back to "folk medicine", the medicine my grandparents practiced. Information is much easier to obtain now with so many holistic organizations, books and web information.

Following years of fighting the traditional medical world, I retired from traditional nursing at 62 years of age, not because I did not need to make money but I knew I could not stay well if I kept working under such stressful conditions. I will say that my body, mind and spirit is younger and healthier than it was 13 years ago. I love the wealth of information available now. I kept studying and working at non medical professions until I could get all 4 of my children through college.

A great deal of the time I was working as a medical professional, I had 2 other jobs just to keep all the college fees paid and keep my children in food and clothing, after my husband died of brain cancer. I have been a Mary Kay Beauty Consultant, A real estate salesperson, A Pampered Chef, a retail sales clerk, a pet sitter, a restaurant hostess, desk clerk and breakfast hostess at a motel, day care and nursery school supervisor, A master bear builder with Build A Bear, an employment counselor, a caterer, an event planner, a health care advocate and many of these jobs were done while I was still working in the traditional medical field as; a med/surg floor supervisor, a critical care nurse, a director of nursing, an administrator of a health care center, a corporate health and wellness nurse, nursing manager of rehab hospital, and each time I went into the hospital/nursing home care field I would again get so stressed out and angry about "no wellness programs for the clients". Is there a record of how many jobs a person has done? I might be like the fellow who changed jobs weekly and wrote a book about it. I would love to write about some of my jobs as they were so much fun and also provided me with extra income. Sometimes the other jobs kept my mental health in good condition.

When I went to Nursing School I was taught very little about wellness but learned a lot about illness and medications. I had to spend a lot of time doing my research; learning how to be well and how to stay well.

I am a very caring person and when I was administrator of a Health Care Center, the government required that I do things I knew were wrong. I had to take the deep heat rub away from a 90 year lady who had used it for over 50 years for her joint pain, instead the Doctor gave her a prescription for a drug that was "approved" and has since been found to be a killer. That is a simple example of what we are doing to our elderly. I used to tell my nurses that when I got to the Nursing Home, when they took my Vicks Vaporub I would have to be restrained. I figured that I was smart enough in the ways of the medical world; I would know how to hide it.

I have kept my own wellness program going and have not had any illness for the past 30+ years with the exception of a few signs of inflammation that can be easily taken care of with a few changes in my program. Some might say that I just had good genes; my mother and father both died before they were my age, one younger sister died several years ago with lots of health problems and my other 2 sisters have lots of health issues, in spite of my insistence for better wellness programs. I have to be very careful advising my family because they have medical professional that they trust.

It is ok to trust your medical professional if he/she allows you to question him and if you will go home after the visit and check out all the instructions that have been given you and check any prescriptions that has been recommended for side effects and natural alternatives before you get them at the pharmacy. If you have a good pharmacist he/she can advise you. Prescriptions, in my opinion should only be used in an emergency until you can assist you body in getting well. If your physician cannot help you **be well**, go somewhere else for your care.

For many years now I have spent 4-6 hours a day doing research and studying holistic medicine. I live on a small acreage with many rescued animals: 14 dogs, 3 cats, a mini mule, a horse, a pygmy goat, a hen and a rooster. I treat my animals well and almost never have to see the vet. I spend some time each day writing wellness plans for people who have developed health problems. Very few people talk about a wellness program until they already have health issues.

Chapter Two

A wellness plan

Here is a list of about 20 things I think everyone should do to achieve optimal wellness: (More info on each point later). I hope I have written this in a way that it will appeal to all age groups and male and female alike.

1. **Find a health care advocate or coach that you trust to help you:** it is so important to have someone help you. The old barn raisings were so much fun and everything got done so fast because people worked together. If the farm family in the community needed a new barn, everyone came together to build him a barn. You might be just doing dishes without help, someone comes to help. The job becomes fun and it is not done just twice a fast but probably 3 times as fast. By the way, I wish I could see some more barn raisings, I think it would make our world a better place. I love projects where people work together. If you have someone to assist you it will give you support and everything will get done faster.

2. **Clean up your diet and environment, this will include getting rid of everything in your house that is toxic to your health, and also includes; stop smoking, if you smoke, your health advocate can help;** You will feel so much better when you throw out the old to bring in the new. It is like starting fresh, or like throwing out your old rusting broken tools and getting all new ones. I have an enormous sweet tooth; the thing that is hardest for me to give up is sweets. I try to satisfy my sweet tooth by taking a bite of dried fruit when I feel the need to have sugar. Be aware that none of us eat healthy all the time but we need to know how to correct our program when we do "mess up".

3. **Find out what supplements you need for your wellness, all programs should include: a quality multi vitamin/mineral supplement, an omega oil, and coenzyme Q10. MSM is another product most people need and most everyone needs, probiotic. Other supplements will be discussed later.** When you read all the resources I give you, you will read some research and decide what your body needs so it can function at its best. There are always new discoveries also. There has been lots of recent research on the Amazon rainforest herbs and I added maca and the camu camu berry to my daily routine as soon as I saw all the research. I was so happy when they did the research and found that cacao; the real chocolate is such a great thing for our wellness.

4. **Develop your exercise program, you may use your own knowledge or hire a trainer for a few lessons.** It is my opinion that health clubs and gyms are a waste of money, but some people find them useful. You can use the money you spend one month at the club and purchase all the equipment you need at home. You may need a friend though to give you emotional support, so invite someone to come every few days for a cup of coffee or a cup of tea and do a little jumping on the mini trampoline or walk. If you have a close neighbor you like, talk to him/her about doing some exercise with you and maybe laugh with you too. There are also some very good computer/TV interactive programs for exercise.

5. **Find a physician that will listen to you and help you with your optimal wellness program and work with you to delete as many prescription medications as possible. If you have prescriptions, read all the literature to make certain you know all the side effects to look for while you are taking it.** I have so many examples of abuse of prescription drugs that I don't know where to begin. Some of the worst in my mind are the drugs for gurd or indigestion. I know someone who was taking the little purple pill for years; it is supposed to be taken only a few weeks at the most. The physician wondered why the patient's bones had almost been deleted and why her vitamin levels were so low. He either did not know or did not care that the little purple pill kept interfering with her body's ability to make use of all those vitamins especially calcium and B12, Calcium and

vitamin D were added to her medications but she is still taking the "little purple pill", what do you think is happening to the supplements, nothing. Now both a physician and a pharmacist are making a mistake. Did they even read the little insert that comes with the drug? I admit that some of this happens because the drug can be purchased over the counter now, but she took it years before she started buying it over the counter.

6. **Make your surroundings peaceful and a place indoors and outdoors that can be used for meditation, relaxation and reading, learn the art of Qigong and practice it or one of the other Chinese breathing and exercise programs.** My grandmother always rocked in her rocking chair near a window to relax and worked in her garden, grandpa was never allowed to work in the garden, that was grandma's time to think things out and watch her plants grow, the product of her labors.

   Many years ago I discovered C-span book TV on television on weekends and holidays, I really enjoy it and it gives me an idea about books and authors that I would like to read, I then check them out on Amazon.com to read some of the book and get the price. It also keeps me from purchasing books that I really do not enjoy. I have enjoyed books from the day I learned to read a few words and even though I no longer read much fiction, I enjoy and learn a lot from nonfiction books. The only fiction I have read lately are books that interest my grandchildren, that is a necessity of life.

7. **Purchase water and an air filtration system for your home, if you cannot afford a full house system there are alternatives.** Our air is full of toxic materials and some of the things our bodies will tolerate for a time but you would not wash your clothes in dirty water or use a dirty wash cloth to dry your dishes so do not breathe dirty air or drink water that has poisons added to it. Our lungs are one of the greatest organs we have and what we breathe goes directly into this organ, so clean up your air.

8. **Do gallbladder/kidney cleanse and if you have elimination problems, do a bowel cleanse (information later), there are other cleanses that you may need as you evaluate your conditions.** I have seen people put themselves through surgery instead of doing a simple gallbladder cleanse. If you shower and

clean the outside of your body, why not clean the inside of your body?

9. **Plan a massage, a visit to the chiropractor and get an infrared sauna, etc. If you have a problem check and see if acupuncture, Reiki or another modality will help:** I have not found the research but I know in my own mind that these procedures can add years to your life and life to your years. Just a simple foot massage touches 52 bones and hundreds of nerves, muscles, joints, etc. And your hands, 54 bones, etc, etc, etc, and none of us get enough human touch. Another part of acupuncture is the old fashioned cupping. I like this modality a lot.

10. **Find a source for good fruits and vegetables, organic if possible.** It is so worth it to get good sources for your fruits, vegetables and meats. It is more expensive but the stuff has been raised and handled by loving hands. Organic meat and dairy is important if you can find a good source.

11. **Choose a pet, one that fits your lifestyle; go to the shelter to look at the possibilities.** Even if it is no more than saying good morning to your messy little bird or listening to the purr of that cat, it will add to your wellness. Besides that, you will be saving a life. If you are interested in an animal and have a tendency toward allergies, have someone test you for an allergy to the animal, muscle testing for weakness is a very easy way to test for individual animals.

12. **Select a group of friends and relatives with positive attitudes to socialize with and laugh with:** It is becoming more of a problem in this modern world, even to talk to someone. I am even getting text messages and I will not text! If someone wants to communicate with me they can talk. My granddaughter carries her phone and when she is talking to me, she is texting someone else. I absolutely hate that. How long has it been since you wrote a long letter to someone, or just had a leisurely cup of coffee with a friend or neighbor? Back in the good old days, even when I was working full time and raising 4 children, I frequently had coffee with a neighbor.

13. **Do something nice for someone else every week:** I went to a conference many years ago that I have never forgotten the key-

note speaker, he had a catchy title for his speech: "dipper in my bucket". He spoke about the fact that we carry around a dipper and bucket, when someone does something nice for you or says something nice about you, your bucket gets filled. When you are nice to someone, not only does it fill their bucket but it fills yours too. When someone says something or does something negative to you or you do something negative to someone else the dipper takes from your bucket and theirs. He said that most people were going around with empty buckets, waiting to be filled. It is so easy to fill the bucket but most usually we are just emptying the bucket of someone. My younger kids picked up on the story when I was telling my husband, so frequently, I heard; "Mom don't dip into my bucket." I don't remember the name of the speaker but I daily remember his message. When I look it up on the web, I can find some school programs and work place program with the theme but not the name of my original speaker, back 35 years ago.

14. **Volunteer weekly:** When you do this you are filling lots of buckets and yours will be filled too. If you cannot think of something you would like to volunteer for, call your chamber of commerce and get a list of non profits in your area.

15. **Find a hobby you are passionate about and start it:** you may have to think back into your past to find the hobby you love. I used to do lots of crafts and I would feel sluggish and remember that I had not done a craft in a while so start crafts and I would be very invigorated. When my children were young, I would stay up late at night to embellish their clothing or make more tee shirts. I also had two friends who did the same things so it was even better. I had a friend who did ceramics, sewing, and many other things with me. Our husbands were golfers so you know we had a lot of time with the children to do things together. When you have a spouse who plays golf, you must have a hobby.

16. **Keep a journal or blog:** I don't know if there is anyone out there reading my blog but I enjoy doing it every day. It also keeps a record so I can go back later to track something.

17. **Be patient and forgiving:** Never hold grudges, I used to have this problem but I learned years ago that it did me lots of harm

so I make myself wake up every morning forgiving all who have wronged me. Sometimes this is a very difficult thing to do.

18. **Give yourself opportunity to learn something new daily:** There is so much to learn and so little time. There is a book that I have in my library that is titled, "The know it all" this guy had memorized most of the encyclopedia and liked to add tidbits to all conservation. I am almost that obnoxious because I know a little about so many things. I find everything so interesting!

19. **Have fun; laugh and play every day:** When my children were young, I had a next door neighbor and we played a lot. If the weather was bad and the snow was deep, we and our husbands got together at one of our homes and played table games, while our children played with their dolls or trucks. My youngest sister and I had an ongoing Yahtzee game that continued each time we were together, sometimes we would not see each other for several months but we had to continue the game each time as we visited. This was on going from the time the kids were in play pens until they now have grown children of their own. My grand kids love table games too. Playing for you may be shopping or some other "sport".

20. **Don't procrastinate- start now!** This is probably the most important thing you can do. Some people have problems just getting started at anything. And we need to be finishers too!

You will notice that I did not include a weight loss plan on the list. There are lots of weight loss plans already available and I feel that a good nutrition program without sugar and white flour will keep your weight at a good level. If you are obese, discuss a plan with your health care advocate or your physician. I think the best weight loss comes from being on an anti fungal diet and increasing your exercise intensity and time. If you have a lot of "belly fat'; two things may be causing it, stress and lack of sleep. When you measure your waist line (at the belly button) it should not be more that one half you height; 5 foot tall, 30 inch waist.

I love the idea of eating as close to raw as possible; this is not the habit of most people so is very hard for us to change. Raw food has so many more digestive enzymes. When you eat raw you also need less food and you have not killed the vitamins with heat. When the food is raw you get the benefits of all the vitamins, minerals, enzymes and fiber.

I am unusual because I like for older people to be at the top of their "normal" weight chart, don't try to be too skinny, just be healthy. Maybe I have spent too much time with elderly people but this is my opinion.

Most of these 20 points will help reduce your stress and that is so important. Some studies say that stress could be the cause of most illness. Most experts think that stress is what causes all your belly fat and is so unhealthy, remember that your belly fat measurement should be less than one-half your height; for example 5 foot tall should have waist line of 30 inches or less. There is a lab test to tell you whether or not the inflammation is damaging your health. You can request a CRP lab test.

If you have a problem with sleep try; using your magnesium gel and take a few drops of passion flower just before bed; including in your bed time snack sunflower seeds might help.

Planning your program is like putting together a quilt, there are many pieces to it and you must put them together in the right order then stitch the pieces together to make it strong. You do not want it to fall apart. And you do not want your wellness program to fall apart. Once you build the steps in your program and make them a habit it will be easier, you know about how hard it is to break a habit, good or bad. My sister used to do classes in which they did a quilt in a day; your wellness program will not be put together in a day so have patience.

You can put together this wellness program at any age, but the younger the better.

Chapter Three

Customizing your plan

Every person is different; therefore, every wellness program is customized to fit. There is no "one size fits all" in a wellness program. If your house is like mine I have many, many electrical and computer cords, all different. When I try to charge a new phone, I will probably have to purchase another cord. There is no universal cord; I spend lots of my time trying to find the right connection for things. I feel that way about wellness programs; you have to find the right connectors for your wellness; the correct exercises, the correct supplements and the right modalities.

Everyone has to make his/her own decisions and plan their own program with the assistance of people they love and that love them. It would probably be much easier if we could just put all the stuff in a can and feed it to everyone.

When you have read this and start your plan, write it down in your journal or on your blog. Many people are so into "instant gratification" that they will not follow through with any wellness plans, because it takes time to become well; a happy person with no health issues at all. You can do parts of the program or all that you believe will work in your individual wellness program. Whatever you do will be your choice. We all choose how we live but we also must live with the consequences of our choices. My ideas have changed as research and information has become available and I choose what I add or delete from my program. Dr. Raymond Francis states in his book, "Never be sick again", poor health is not a matter of luck but a matter of choice.

Many times when I have discussed a plan with people they say, "I just do what my doctor says, he knows best." Any good physician would tell you to question everything a provider says and insist they help you **be well**. *Everyone must participate in his/her own wellness plan. You cannot depend on someone else to tell you exactly what to do.*

I have little patience with people who whine and say, 'it's too hard'. In fact, in today's language, I have "zero tolerance" for whiners. Even when my children were young, I did not tolerate whining.

The most important thing you can do is listen to your body. Your body will tell you when you need to change your plan. A few months ago I fell and pulled my hamstring, (I was being unwise and chasing my horse over wet ground) I did a few really wonderful ballet moves, if I were an athlete I would have gone on the "DL" (disabled list) I am an avid 'watcher" of sports so I think a lot in sports terms. It took me a while to recover but with a little change in my program I got through it. During the ordeal and with little exercise, I gained inches in my waist so have the problem of correcting that also.

It takes longer to heal as you get older and also there was the problem of restarting exercising and also recapture my gait, (walking correctly). It is really important to start walking properly as soon as possible because you will get your joints and muscles trained wrong and they will be harmed. When I was nursing manager in the rehab hospital, I learned a lot about the proper gait and how important it is to walk correctly.

The short time I was on the DL made me realize once again that I enjoy being well and plan to stay that way.

When I read my body I found that I needed to treat inflammation from the inside out because I developed an inflamed eye to tell me to get busy and treat for inflammation. Each time that I get inflammation it ends up as a severe dry eye. One of the things I did was double my intake of krill oil and increased my antioxidant intake. I also started watching my sugar intake more closely. I started taking oil of oregano and olive leaf extract. It seemed like a long time but it was really just a couple of weeks until I was well again. It takes a baseball player much longer to recover from a hamstring injury and he is much younger than I. He had all the modalities of modern medicine to assist him in getting well. The reason I got well faster is because of my competitiveness, stubbornness and maybe it was just the necessity.

During the big flu scare, I instructed everyone to take oil of oregano, olive leaf extract, wash with neem soap and keep hands away from the face. Taking more antioxidants and staying hydrated is important. It has been many, many years since I have had an upper respiratory infection or the flu and I never take a flu injection. If I recall it was in the 1980's when I last had a problem.

Dr. Andrew Weil has a complete guide that I like, on his website and in one of his books. In the guide Dr. Weil talks about the anti inflammatory diet and I will give you some of that information later in this book. As I have stated; to check your inflammation and what it is doing to your body, you can have a CRP test run.

Your advocate can be a family member, friend or a hired wellness coach. When she/he helps you clean up your environment, donate what you take out of your house to a shelter or a day care center. I think you should get rid of white sugar, white flour, white rice, most processed foods and artificial sweeteners (keep honey, stevia and sweeteners you find healthy). Anything that has the bad fats in it needs to be thrown out, that includes the fats that are disguised as vegetable oil. Read all the labels. If you want to find out how dangerous artificial sweeteners are, just read the research. I would never put a diet soda in my mouth or anything else that has been sweetened with artificial sweeteners. I had a liquid supplement that I used to just love but the company decided they would add splenda to it and I never took another swallow of it. With that I figured the company was not there to make people healthy but was there to make money. Many years ago I enjoyed reading Prevention magazine, as soon as they started advertising prescription drugs, I decided they had sold out to the drug industry and I would never trust them again. As you realize from my ramblings, I am very opinionated and have a very narrow margin that I allow people or companies to work from.

Restock your shelves with healthy foods, read labels. Get lots of spices, healthy oils, healthy sweeteners, etc. If you use whole fruits instead of juices, you will get more nutrition and less sugar. I no longer use a juicer, I emulsify with my magic bullet a real emulsifier is too expensive to purchase for just one person so I use the bullet and it works fine. If you prefer to juice, that is good but you will receive more calories from the juice than the whole fruit.

Do not ever heat anything in plastic; if you do you will get many, many toxins in your body. I don't even store liquids in plastic because if the container gets warm the plastic gets into your food. I never drink from plastic if I can avoid it. I never put plastic in the microwave. I use the microwave as little as possible because some experts report that the microwaves change the properties of your food, just in case they are correct, I do not use the microwave much. I do not have any plastic in my kitchen excepting when someone brings it in. I also do not let aluminum foil touch my food, I will place parchment paper over the food and put the foil over the paper when I need to place foil on something. I think the foil emits toxins when it touches some of the foods especially foods that contain acids.

It is not surprising that my generation has so many health problems; we were taught that margarine was good for you; liver was a necessary food, etc. This was also the time they started pre mixing everything and adding lots of preservatives and food colorings.   When my patients in the health care center refused their required servings of liver, I would secretly cheer because I knew how many toxins they were avoiding. Liver is full of the toxins the animal has filtered out of its system via the liver, and we eat it. We were taught that liver was the best source of iron, but we know that there are lots of other sources and we do not need to eat the toxic livers of animals to keep our iron level normal. One good source, spinach. I know that spinach is good for me, I do not like spinach, and so I put baby spinach in with my salad greens and get it that way or emulsify it with other vegetables.

Most of us are dehydrated, it is so important for our wellness to drink plenty of liquids. I do not promote the idea that everyone needs a certain quantity of water,

I think each of us is different and the foods we are consuming differ. Everyone is different so be sure you are never thirsty at all and your skin is never dry.

Research your supplements: start with a resource you trust and your health care advocate, begin with the multiple vitamin/mineral, it can be a liquid, a powder or a capsule, I prefer liquid or powder. Any time you can get a supplement in liquid, drops, spray or skin gel it will get directly into your system. If you get a capsule or tablet, leave one in water and see if it dissolves in 3 hours, if it does not it will do you little good. One 87 year old lady was given an iron tablet, the physician thought she really needed badly, I placed it in warm water, 2 days later it was still almost completely whole. Do you think she was getting any good from that tablet or was it just expensive bowel movement?

Everyone needs an omega 3 fatty acid, this can be fish or krill oil in gel form or in a liquid or a capsule, years ago all winter I would pour cod liver oil in the orange juice of my children, it is easier to take now. I take an omega 3,6,9 and krill oil. Coenzyme Q10 is made by your body to repair and energize your cells until you are around 40 years old then it needs replacement, I suggest 100 mgm a day, if you have high blood pressure you probably need 100 mgm. 3 times a day. There are lots of prescription drugs that deplete the coQ10 too. MSM is a substance that you need to investigate; it is used in allergies, for treating intestinal parasites, useful for joint problems, including arthritis and many other things. I like the supplement, resveratrol made from the grape. If you have family history of some diseases this is a necessary supplement, one example is diabetes.

I think all of us need a quality antioxidant, drink noni juice, goji berry juice, mangosteen, acai berry or the one I take; Zamu (a blend from the rain forest), www. freddie.amazonherbs.net, I also drink noni, goji and acai. And I eat a lot of blueberries, I was really happy when they started drying them and cranberries too.

Read information on alpha lipoic acid, especially if you have blood sugar problems or a family history of blood sugar problems. If you do not eat a lot of raw fruits and vegetable, you will need some digestive enzymes. Probiotics keep your good bacteria in your digestive system so that all your vitamins and minerals can work; if you have taken antibiotics you have a big need for the probiotics. Your regiment should deal with any health problems you have. I have no prescription drugs in my house.

In Dr. Weil's anti inflammatory diet he has lots of fresh fruits and vegetables. He includes more pasta than my body will tolerate but most of his suggestions, I agree with. He is a real expert on herbs, it would be good for you to visit his website and/or read his books.

There are lots of herbs and foods that can be a substitute for prescriptions and there are no side effects. I will list resources near the end of the book. I will also list experts on each major disease.

In my opinion prescription drugs became a much bigger problem when two things happened; drug companies were allowed to hire just anyone to sell their products to medical practitioners, many years ago you had to be a pharmacist to sell prescriptions. The other thing that happened was companies were allowed to sell drugs on TV. You know the popular ads that say, "ask your doctor if this drug would be good for you." I like the one that says, if you decide to commit suicide after taking XYZ, call your doctor immediately. Or when it says that the most usual side effect is; heart attack. I know they do not say exactly that but it is close.

Most people need to supplement with vitamin D and Magnesium if there is not enough in their multi vitamin/mineral. I believe B12, sublingual or spray is important. All the old country doctors I knew, when I was young, gave a lot of "magic shots", everyone received a vitamin B12 injection, and felt much better, it also made them love their doctors and visit the doctor every month. Way back in the 60's I knew an old country doctor that had an office full of different colored baby aspirin and a lot of B12, he was a great diagnostician so knew when someone just needed to be listened to and who was really ill.

Recent research shows that most people are deficient in B12, magnesium and vitamin D, most everyone thought for years that we got these products in our food and sunshine, food from most sources have been depleted of a great many vitamins and minerals, and we no longer use the sun without sun screen, I never use sunscreen, I limit the sun by how my skin feels and looks. When I see someone who wears sunglasses all the time, I want to tell them that they are doing something very wrong for their wellness. I think you should wear sunglasses only when the sunlight is making you squint your eyes. A hat, cap or an old fashioned bonnet will work well when you are out in the sun. This is my opinion only but I have read a lot of research that agrees with me.

Make a habit of drinking teas, I have had to teach myself to drink tea and some teas, I just plain do not enjoy, so I drink the ones I enjoy. When I was young we never had tea in our old farmhouse so I think it is hard sometimes to change your tastes, to enjoy something you never learned to enjoy as a young person. It is good though that we never had sodas so never got the soda habit. When I was in Nursing School and worked the night shift, I had not gotten used to tea, coffee or colas so had to learn to drink a cola when I was working the night shift, just for a pick-me-up in order to tolerate the soda, I had to add a little ice cream to it.

When you are developing your exercise program, simple is better. The things I think you need are: stretching bands (sometimes a physical therapist will get you some very cheap), a balance ball, a rebounder and some simple weights (if you don't have weights, use plastic bags containing rice or beans). A rebounder will help your lymph system and keeps all your fluids in your body active. If you decide to hire a trainer, tell him/her that you want as little equipment as possible. I also use a Pilates bench but it is not necessary. There are at least 5 conditions that physical activity can reduce your risk for; heart disease, obesity, stroke, diabetes and fractures. Exercise will also help you sleep better and give you more energy.

Yoga may be something you want to do, it is said to improve many aspects of your life including; creating a sense of well being and calm and improve your circulation and concentration. If you are interested in learning yoga, you may want to check out websites and www.youtube.com to learn how to do yoga.

You also may want to learn Qigong, start on www.youtube.com and see if it is something you want to learn how to do, I am going to become a master of Qigong.

Walking is important for everyone. Measure how well you are doing on flexibility and strength by doing your every day chores. If you cannot put your pants on, standing in the middle of the room, you need to do more to improve your balance. If you cannot carry a 40 or 50 pound bag of something across the room, increase strength exercises, etc. If you cannot bend and reach the floor, your flexibility exercises need to be better.

A few years ago I went to check out a local health club, the receptionist/sales person, ask me what I wanted from a program and I told her; I want to carry my horse food (50 lbs.) from the car to the barn, I wanted to lift my 5 gallon of water that is in a glass container and place it on the dispenser on the cabinet and I wanted not to wobble when I put my clothes on in the middle of the room. She really did not know anyone had goals like that.

Be an explorer and explore all your options when it comes to exercise and movement. There are so many things you can do so find things you can really enjoy. Some people get a lot of their exercise just dancing. When I was a young person, I did square dance and it was exercise and fun.

Finding a holistic health professional may be a problem, it is in my part of the world, some family physicians can be taught to help you. If your physician says you do not need supplements, just eat well; get out of his office as soon as possible. Everyone knows that the soil is so depleted that the carrot your grandparents ate would need to be replaced by many more now. A compounding pharmacy or a health food store may be able to give you some suggestions on how to find a "user friendly" health care professional.

I wrote an article and did some speeches on, "How to Hire a Doctor". You should interview your medical professionals just as you would if you were hiring

a maid or baby sitter. When you find your provider, request that they order saliva testing at a compounding pharmacy for hormone level testing; a place for chelating heavy metals and any other lab tests that will help you make decisions about your health. If you cannot afford intravenous chelating, there are oral supplements for chelating but it takes longer. There is a product from nutritional research made by, Dr. Garry Gordon called: BC 1, that I like very much. There are probably lots *of other modalities to assist you but I am not aware of others. A large number of people have abnormal levels of thyroid and other hormones, so testing hormone levels should be one of the first things a physician will do. Some of the norms for hormones are not good for everyone, this is another thing that is not a "one size fits all" so you must explore what is correct for you.*

When my daughter got out of college and started living in an apartment, she started having seizures; I had a very difficult time finding a physician that did chelating for heavy metals. We finally found one and she did the oral chelating because we could not afford the intravenous treatments. You also need a lab that will test your blood for fungus. If you are thought to be diabetic, be certain that your physician does more lab tests than the fasting blood sugar, there are several ways of measuring what the blood sugar levels are doing to your body, one that I know about is the one that measures the blood sugar that is attached to your hemoglobin molecule. Do your own research and find out the tests and treatments that are available. Modern medicine has so many things available that can assist you in knowing what to do to be well.

Prepare relaxation places: one in the house and one outdoors. You need a place in the house that is very relaxing and peaceful. I like a comfortable chair with a reading light and a table for writing, reading, doing brain exercises and meditating. Outdoors should be a place where you can get your 30 minutes of sunshine and also a shady place to read, listen to music, do puzzles and brain exercises and write in your journal. Brain exercises can be as simple as puzzles or games. I love "brain games".

For relaxing music you can go to www.youtube.com and find anything you like. There are lots of resources on that web address, also many exercise and stretching programs. I got my first deep breathing exercise from youtube. It is amazing how cheap and easy it is to access almost anything you want in the way of info; videos or audio. I am very fond of Qigong for breathing and general improvement of health.

Near your outside space should be your garden; I try to increase my garden space every year, a water fountain a birdfeeder, etc. I also have a birdfeeder in my dining room window, watching my cardinals during ice or snow is really great. You may start your garden with just some large pots and extend it as you want, it will depend on your space and your interest in gardening. I love to get the wonderful fruits and vegetables from my little garden that are free of pesticides. The best way to start sometimes is with an herbal garden.

Having a good air and water filtration system in your home is critical. If there are no funds for a full house system, start with a Britta pitcher and a small air filter for your bedroom or the room where you spend most of your time. I have very limited funds so I have a small air filtration system for my living room and one for my bedroom. My water filtration system is one that I was given because the friend did not like it. Everyone knows that I am not going to refuse any regift if I can use it. My wish list contains a whole house air and water filtration system.

I think everyone should have a pet if at all possible, it may be a dog, a cat, a bird etc. there is lots of research to say that just petting your cat or dog or talking to your bird will improve your immune system and lower your blood pressure. Your pet can also be a very inexpensive psychiatrist, someone to tell your troubles to and confide in any time you need to unload.

One year after my husband died, my house burned, I had 2 kids in college, one in high school and one in junior high. The Sunday after my house burned, my dog was replaced by a Border collie puppy, given to my children. What to do with a puppy when I had no house, we managed and that Border collie, Oreo, became my psychiatrist, an inexpensive one. I could tell him my problems, "fuss" at him, talk out my decisions; all in all he was probably the best thing that happened to me. Even though I thought having him to care for was the worst thing that could happen at the time.

Pray and be thankful, this includes having a forgiving spirit. When you pray or meditate you make great improvements in you emotional health and your goal to "being well". If you do not have a forgiving spirit, you will neither be well or happy.

There is several different oxygen therapies that I think could be a component in any wellness program, following an illness. Hyperbaric oxygen and EWOT, a program in which you exercise with oxygen going into your system, are two of the programs I like. This is especially necessary if you have had a stroke or have a neurological disease. Find out if there are programs such as these in your area and take advantage of them. I see oxygen bars now but have not tried one yet, I plan to soon, just to see how it is supposed to work. Lots of these things are just a way to get your money so be aware of the person who is waiting just to get you money.

One of the greatest things you can do for your health is, LAUGH! Laugh every day, find someone to laugh with or laugh at a funny movie. When you laugh, you not only lift your spirit, you exercise a lot of your body. I have a few movies that just thinking about them makes me laugh. They are on old tapes so have to find a way to change them to DVDs. If you are feeling down, call a friend or relative who can pull you up or find something to laugh at, don't feel guilty about playing. Play should be a part of every day. So many people who grew up when I did forgot to play after they became an adult. Play and laughter are very inexpensive too.

If you have health issues, do some research and find the things that will make you well.

Getting rid of all the heavy metals in your system that is keeping you from being well is very important. Also important is cleansing your digestive tract, liver, gallbladder and kidneys. There are cleanses you can purchase; I get the recipes and do my own. You can find information from the expert, Dr Hulda Clark, these cleanses are necessary to do as soon as possible.

If you need a weight reduction program put it together with the assistance of your physician and your health advocate. Choose a program and start it, sometimes you do better on a weight loss program if you have a partner. Choose someone who has a great attitude and is fun to be around.

If you have had heart problems and your physician has not told you to take these supplements, he is far behind in his research. The supplements that are absolutely necessary to re energize your heart are: D-Ribose, CoenzymeQ10, Fish oil, Magnesium and l-carnitine. All the resources I read, talk about the importance of these supplements to make you well. Magnesium pills are rather large and you may be more pleased with the gel to rub on your skin. It is a good idea to rub it on at bedtime because it also helps sleep. A good cardiologist will give large doses of all these supplements until he/she has you feeling "top notch".

See if your problem can be helped with acupuncture, I believe massage and an infrared sauna is very important, they both help alleviate the problems of getting rid of toxins and relieve stress. They make you feel good too; I think everyone should get a weekly massage and an infrared sauna at least every three months, if you can afford it.

Way back when I went to nursing school, we were taught that no one went to sleep at night without a good back rub. That back rub many times eliminated the need for sleeping pills .Acupressure and aroma therapy are additional therapies that make you feel good, when I massaged my sister's hands and feet with aroma oils it makes us all feel better. A foot and hand massage does not take much time or energy and can do wonders for even the ones of us who have ultimate wellness.

Before you use any of the modalities, interview the practitioner and if you do not like him or her, get another one. Don't visit any practitioner that you do not like and anyone who does not let you participate in your care.

Music therapy can also do wonders for us, at this moment; I have 14 dogs lying at my feet and throughout the living room, taking wonderful naps while listening to classical music. I call that music therapy.

If you have anyone in the area who does NAET or other sensitivity testing, get rid of your sensitivities, NAET con be found on the internet and it will give you a list of trained people in your area. I went for the training without really believing it would really work, because it looks like voodoo but I found that it worked. There are also some home test kits; Dr. Pescatore has a test kit on his website that I am going to try.

Two other modalities that you might want to research are EFT and Reflexology. Both have helped people who have health problems or aches and pains. I was introduced to EFT when I met an acquaintance I had not seen in a while and *asked him about his chronic back pain, he told me he learned tapping (EFT) and no longer had pain. I thought this might be helpful to others so I ordered all the materials so I could have the knowledge. I frequently follow leads like that to enable me to find procedures or modalities that will assist people and animals in being well.*

When I was trying to keep my family well, I learned NAET and Reflexology; I also researched the different oxygen therapies and Chinese herbal medicine.

I am working to become a master of Qigong because that appears to be the best overall program for my wellness. Energy healing is something I just recently started learning and Reiki. I am also studying King Institute's method of using TKM, you can find out more about TKM if you look at the website www.kinginstitute.org. I am always trying to find every method I can for self-healing. In this age of electronics you can access information so easy and so fast and you have to stay aware of information as it changes. Explore and investigate, that is my method of learning.

People used to wear garlic and onion to ward of infections, this is no longer acceptable but it works; now we can get it in our food and in supplements. For any infection the onions, garlic and oil of oregano continue to be the answer but we have more effective delivery systems now and more user friendly too.

Chapter Four

Setting goals

Don't plan to do your program quickly, proceed slowly but surely taking each step. Don't get discouraged when you do not achieve ultimate wellness the first week or the first month. It takes time to reverse the illness we have invited to live in our bodies. You will begin to feel changes and it is a good idea to keep track of all your changes in your journal. Remember that this is for a lifetime. Sometimes you will feel worse before you start feeling better.

I am a goal setter and hope you are too. Set some goals and write down steps to get to your goals. I even set small goals such as writing my blog with "no misspellings", reaching a goal gives me such pleasure that it encourages me to set all kinds of goals. There is a website called "Thrillionaires" it gives you a space to write down those things you want to accomplish. When my children were young, I encouraged them to make goal posters; they were surprised when they had reached those goals.

Many years ago I spent the summer in Arizona, caring for the horse ranch of my son. I had to set goals so I set such goals as; get the horses fed and watered before the temperature reached 100 degrees, keeping my puppy from leaving his little tootsie rolls in the house and getting my exercise in the pool before the water began to boil. It was not ideal but the goal setting helped me measure the progress of my day and kept everything from being boring. I absolutely hate to hear someone say they are bored, there is so much to do and such little time.

It is important to know that you are going to fail, at some time, when you do, laugh, talk to yourself and get on track again.

Chapter Five

Piecing it all together

I will repeat the steps to the program:

- **Enlist someone to be your health advocate, someone you like:**
  If you have the funds available you may want to hire a wellness
  coach but be certain that it is someone you like. It is always better to have someone to talk things over with and make decisions
  easier.

- **Make a list of friends and relatives you can count on to help
  you, people to play and laugh with;** You will add to this list
  as you come in contact with people. Most likely the list will be
  made up of;, neighbors, friend and relatives. It is more fun to do
  things with someone else; it is hard to have fun alone.

- **Get rid of all the toxins in your house and in your body:** This
  will take a while and it is important to start on this little chore
  quickly. It may take you a while just to figure out what is toxic
  to your body. Checking to see what you are sensitive to, is a step
  toward finding what is toxic to you..

- **Find a holistic physician or any physician that will work with
  you on your plan:** Your present health care provider may be
  willing to work with you; all you can do is ask.

- **Schedule appointments for massage, learning Qigong, getting an infrared sauna, chiropractor, Reiki, physician, someone who does acupuncture, etc.** This can be so much fun and
  interesting.

- **Put together products you are going to use for your cleanse, then start to cleanse:** Most of these have to be done when you can be out of circulation for a few days. I usually plan on 2 days of "yucky" stuff, but you will feel good after they are completed. If you are working it will have to be done when you can be off work for a couple of days.

- **Go to the shelter for a pet:** You need a couple of people with you when you do this so you will discuss the pros and cons and choose the right pet. Remember that this is a decision that is permanent and needs to be thought through.

- **Decide on the place you are going to perform your volunteer hours, something you can really feel good about doing;** You may already be doing this if so just evaluate what you are doing and see if it is the thing you want to do instead of something someone else wants you to do. If time permits you may want to spend more time volunteering. I found a church group that would let me go with them on a couple of disaster mission trips.

- **Make a list of people you want to do nice things for and start:** This can be a fun, fun, little job. Remember it can fill their bucket and fill yours at the same time. Start filling buckets!

- **Download music for relaxation, deep breathing, exercises etc.** Go through lots of music and choose a few pieces, you may want to change it later on. I went to www.utube.com and wrote "music for relaxation" and listened to a lot before I decided on a few pieces. I have found that it is difficult for me to do meditation and relax, since I have kept so busy for so many years, it was difficult beyond words to just sit and do nothing. I decided that it was important for my wellness and taught myself to sit quietly, relax and meditate. If you have a problem getting relaxed put a few drops of the herb, passion flower to your cup of tea. It will give you an amazing calm and in turn add to your wellness.

- **Prepare your "nest" indoors and outdoors, for relaxation:** This is something that you will want to evaluate at times and take away or add to so that you can benefit the most from it. I had a physician tell me several years ago that he had a can of indoor air and a can of outdoor air in his office and there was no difference, I beg to disagree, most of the time the indoor air is much more toxic, especially since our homes are much more insulated and no fresh air gets in and less stale air gets out, that is the reason for air filtration systems. Another possibility for relaxation is a mud bath or some aroma therapy.

- **Shop for your supplements at health food store or online:** start out with your basics then add to and take away as you do more and more research.

- **Put together your menus and purchase groceries that will add to your wellness:** Don't eat something just because it is good for you, be certain to plan menus using food you love and food that is good for you at the same time and do be willing to try new things.

- **Get your journal and start your blog:** You may already do this but I highly recommend that you journal and blog.

- **Start your medicine cabinet products,** decide what products you want to keep in your medicine cabinet and start purchasing them.

- **Build your exercise program also some brain activities and reading materials;** Collect puzzles, games and other things that will challenge your brain. The exercises you plan to do need to be in a convenient place. I used to start my day with the "crypto quote" in the newspaper every morning.

- **Make a list of your drugs so you can start replacing them with naturals that have no side effects.** If your health care provider is not interested in helping you do this, go somewhere else and find someone who will help you. You and your advocate can do the research and do it with his/her supervision.

- **Find air and water filtration systems:** I think that whole house water and air filtration systems have to be on everyone's wish list. If we are taking hot showers in water that is full of toxins such as fluorine, it cannot be healthy.

- **Put your wellness plan into action—Do IT NOW- DO IT NOW**

I think your daily routines would look something like this:

- Stretching exercise early, maybe just a couple of toe touches and "reach for the sky" a couple of times as soon as you get out of bed

- Say out loud, "I forgive all who have wronged me", and then think about whose bucket you will fill today.

- Healthy breakfast and take supplements

- Other exercise of some kind during the day

- A time to relax, maybe only a few minutes, meditate/prayer and relaxing music

- Exercise your mind, as time permits

- Spend some time in the sunshine if possible

- Healthy lunch and dinner

- Write in journal/blog either early in am or late in the evening.

- If you are working a 10 hour day and have children, you can work in your wellness program throughout the day. Time management is very important when you are working and caring for children and it is even more important for a mother to work her wellness program into the daily routine.

When I was working at a job in which I had to assist people in getting jobs, I made it clear to them that the best way to get a job was by networking. I continue to believe that networking is important and at this time in my life some of it is social networking, using the computer to blog, twitter, facebook, etc.

I also think it is important for most of us to take classes to learn new things. I take classes online, since I am almost "housebound", I do not leave the animals I have rescued very often. I am usually involved in at least two classes at all times. I also take advantage of a lot of free newsletters I like, on line.

Earlier in my life I took classes at the community college and attended seminars on anything I was interested in, I even had a class in flower arranging and a class in scrap booking. When I was administrator of a health care center, I went to all the seminars; drug seminar for the nurses, activity director workshops, social services workshops and nutrition workshops. I attended some seminars on music therapy and recreational therapy. I learned something useful every time I went to a lecture, a seminar or a workshop.

Whatever job I choose to do, I try to become an expert. A few years ago a Dr. in Texas called and requested that I work with NAET to help a child nearby who had autism. I had never had opportunity to be involved with anyone diagnosed with autism, so I began to read everything I could find and found every site I could on the internet. I told the family that I would be happy to work with them to eliminate his allergies if they started cleaning up his nutrition and started him on a really good liquid supplement. The story was a success as the child improved a great deal.

I tell this story to let you know that I want to be an expert on everything and of course, that is not possible but I will do my best to learn everything I can about everything I am involved with.

Chapter Six

Resources

I am going to give you a list of resources, I rarely agree completely with any expert, I take what I need and believe and store the rest of the information. Usually I find several resources that agree before I take the information and deal with it. If I want to try a new supplement, I get the research that has been done on it and find several sources that agree. If you do not use a computer, go to the library or find a friend or relative who can assist you in looking up some of these websites and books.

Using a computer certainly has enhanced my life and I think it will enhance yours too. When I learned the computer, years ago, I decided since I knew where the on and off button was located, I could not mess up too badly.

In order to really rely on what someone says, you have to evaluate whether or not it is hype to sell something or is it really good reliable information. I am not a very trusting person so I don't believe sales talk. I can't sell because, I feel guilty if I am making money by selling something, even though I believe in it completely. I developed such a negative feeling about sales when I had so many 'door to door' sales people when my kids were growing up. Oh, what hype, I heard.

I love teaching and training but do not love selling, even though I have done some in my past life. Years ago when I was selling real estate, when I had a deal, my broker would ask me, if the people begged me long enough that I agreed to sell them the property. When someone bought property from me they knew they got a good deal and were not being cheated.

Youtube or Ihealthtube has lots of information in the form of videos and they are usually short. When you watch a video evaluate whether or not they are selling something.

www.ihealthtube.com www.youtube.com I use these resources every day, for fun, for information and I find them so interesting.

www.amazon.com when I find something I want, I always check the price against the price on www.amazon.com and www.borders.com

www.swansonsvitamins.com a good source for supplements and also has lots of research articles available to read. This company is very reliable and also very inexpensive

www.seagate.com they grow their own olive leaf extract and does all the processing. They have very good supplements; they even grow their own vegetables and make them into capsules, carrots, broccoli, etc. I would love to visit this place, because they are so dedicated to their products and their quality control.

www.ourhealthcoop I purchase lots of supplements from this company. They are good and very reasonably priced.

www.bioactivenutrients.com is a source of information and supplements.

www.probiotics12.com a great resource for probiotics. There are lots of places to purchase probiotics, you just have to do the research and find the company you want to work with.

www.knowthecause.com Doug Kaufman's website, I do not always agree with him but he has some good information. He does have a good anti fugal diet that I like.

www.restandrepair.com a refreshing way of getting extra oxygen.

www.bioinnovations.net Dr Becker is a good source of information and supplements. This is a physician that has been ill with cancer and he loves to teach others about supplements.

www.wilsonsyndrome.com a must for people who have thyroid problems. You can learn about why so many people are undiagnosed with thyroid when they have lots of symptoms and need help.

www.prevagen.com Mark Underwood, a scientist developed this memory supplement. I like it!

www.drgregemerson.com This Dr. is a real advocate of wellness.

www.mercola.com a resource for lots of holistic health information, Dr. Mercola was about the first internet physician to put together information on nearly everything. You can listen to Dr. Mercola and learn so much. He has so much information on his website and he has written "Take control of your health" which is very good. I take his krill oil as my omega 3 supplement.

www.healingtheeye.com a resource for treatments to keep the eyes healthy, I was so happy to find the information on this website because my vision is so important to me, my husband was blind for a year before he died so I know how important vision is for quality of life.

www.nutritionalresearch.net I use this homeopathic eye health, another aid for my eye health.

www.vitality101.com this is Dr. Tietelbaum's website and he is the very best expert on chronic fatigue and fibromyalgia, this is a physician who has "been there done that" He had fibromyalgia when he was in medical school and looked for the answers that he now shares with everyone.

www.huldaclark.com This physician puts together the cleanse recipes and has lots of information on the webpage also; see curezone.com

www.drwhitaker.com a great physician with lots of knowledge, also has a wellness center in California, anyone who can afford it should go to his clinic for a complete health check. This is the ultimate in diagnosing and treating illness with natural medicine.

www.drweil.com a holistic physician in Arizona, lots of knowledge, is also an expert on herbs, I really love to read the things that Dr. Weil writes and he has so much knowledge about Chinese medicine and herbs.

www.russellblaylock.com An expert on many things, a very good resource for information on toxins and cancer, this is one of the most knowledgeable physicians that I have heard and read.

www.drstengler.com I think this physician is very knowledgeable. I can spend days reading the book he has written on natural health.

www.drsinatra.com a heart specialist and author, he really cares about people. He even takes his dog to his office, that alone would make me love him. If I develop a heart or circulatory problem, this is my guy.

www.drperlmutter.com a brain specialist, if I had a neurological problem, I would hurry to his clinic. He is the first person I started reading when my daughter began to have seizures.

www.drshealy.com a great natural health researcher

www.drpescatore.com has lots of info on fibromyalgia, allergies etc.

www.colecenter.com an endless supply of info on holistic health, if you have time to listen to almost any interviews on any health subject, go to this website.

www.healthybynature.com radio shows on health and old shows in archives you can listen to on many, many subjects. If you want information on a cd you can get it here.

www.sunfoods.com is a resource for natural cacao, goji, acai etc. David Wolfe is the nutrition expert on this site and he is really great. I get my Maca here and it is a super, super food. I would like to spend a week with David Wolfe just to "pick his brain" on nutrition and raw foods.

www.nicabm.com mind and body connections

www.ultrawellness.com Dr. Mark Hyman nutrition program, I really like this physician, he has a lot of info on videos also.

www.usingneem.com The many uses of neem, go to this website just for information. I first discovered this website when my friend's old dog had mange. Neem has so many uses and next year I hope to grow my own neem trees.

www.freddiemema.blogspot.com I blog almost every day about what is going on in my life.

www.memaswellness.homestead.com

www.freddie@amazonherbs.net

www.curenaturalcancro.com Dr. Simoncini an oncologist that I would consult if I had cancer. He treats cancer with the all natural approach and has lots of info on the website. The other cancer clinic I like is Dr. Gonzalez' clinic in New York

www.cancerfightingstrategies.com a complete list of natural ways to cure cancer, this webpage has more info than you probably want to know but it is great.

American Holistic Health Association to see holistic articles on all subjects

The Green Pharmacy is a very good resource, written by Dr. Duke, this book is worthwhile if you are trying to replace some medications with natural cures.

Dr. Bernie Seigel is a great oncologist who uses holistic medicine. I really like this guy, recordings of his books helped me so much almost 20 years ago when I was in intensive care nursery with a grandson, just listening to his audios and videos is a great pleasure, he has written books too.

Dr. Carolyn Dean is an expert on women's health and magnesium, a website called jigsaw health

Dr. Mary Ann Block is an expert on adhd and also depression. She has several books and does free seminars. Her center is in the Fort Worth, Texas area.

Jordan Rubin is a great resource for digestive problems. This is a physician who almost died and found his own cure. He loves to share his info and the first book of his that I got was free, just because he wants people to know about digestive problems and cures.

Dr. Paul Blanc, M.D. has lots of information on toxins but it is a very scientific book and is hard to read

Dr. Cass Ingram is a great resource for natural cures, his book "Lifesaving Cures" should be in everyone's home, I am never without his oil of wild oregano; he can spice up your health with ancient herbs and spices.

Dr. Patrick Quillin is an expert on nutrition and cancer, he also promotes sinus cleansers. His wife also has a vegetarian cookbook.

Dr, Sherry A. Rogers has several books on wellness a great holistic MD with lots of knowledge and has info on pain management

Dr. Elizabeth Lipski-digestive wellness is her subject and she is very knowledgeable.

Dr. Garry Gordon, a wonderful wellness advocate, loads of info and I agree with him almost always

Frank Jordan is another very knowledgeable person on the subject of wellness and promotes www.nsc24.com he is an expert on beta glucans. He has a radio show: Healthy, Wealthy and Wise that is broadcast on line.

If you are interested in any of the Energy Healing Modalities:

- For TKM; www.kinginstitute.org is a very unusual treatment concerning emergency medicine
- Spring Forest Qigong by Chunyi Lin is the qigong that I practice
- Donna Eden healing energy is a very good resource that I use and am learning from these DVDs
- Tai Chi for beginners is a place to start with tai chi, mine came from Tai Chi productions
- Reiki: Judith Conroy is the place to start, I think, Chikara Reiki do, is the DVD that I started watching
- There are usually reflexology and acupuncture practitioners in the areas now so research them locally

This is a list of things to start out with and I encourage you to try the energy healing modalities.

This is just a partial list of the resources I use and if you need additional information on any of them I will be glad to help. You may be overwhelmed with all this info but I want everyone to have lots of choice for information.

I no longer want to over stimulate my brain so I let other people do all the science stuff, I then read enough of their work to make up my mind on what I should do.

Chapter Seven

Some of Mema's Routines

Every Day:

- Always stretch in the morning before I do anything
- Verbally forgive everyone who has wronged me.
- Always eat breakfast
- Always take my supplements
- Always plan a snack in the afternoon
- I try to exercise as I watch TV and run with my dogs
- Write in my blog and my journal every day
- Connect with friends or family every day
- Do Qigong and Energy Healing exercises
- Spend some time exercising my brain and meditating
- If there is sunshine, spend at least 30 minutes outdoors
- Always spend time researching and learning
- If there is sun, I spend as much time as possible in the sunshine

Everyone has their own likes, dislikes and ideas, but I am going to share some of the things I eat and do,

I usually have one of two breakfasts:

Old fashioned oatmeal with a few added things to make it healthier and add more to my wellness. Some of the things I add; Salba, freshly ground Flaxseed, raisins or other dried fruit, a few goji berries, honey, unsweetened coconut, nuts (pecans, almonds, or walnuts) and top it off with a tablespoon of butter. I sometimes add cinnamon but I don't really like cinnamon in my oatmeal even though cinnamon is one of those spices that keep your blood sugar levels normal. It also lowers bad cholesterol.

About 2 mornings a week I will have eggs and Oatnut toast, I am one of those persons who believe coffee is good for you if you do not drink an excessive amount. I have coffee every morning and drink some Zamu and either goji berry or noni juice. Even though some experts disagree with me, I drink raw milk and enjoy it very much. Another juice that I like is pomegranate juice.

Sometime during the day I drink a smoothie with a few things added: cacao, ocean greens, maca, bee pollen, acai and I sweeten it with raw honey.

Some of my favorite foods: sweet potato, broccoli, cabbage, Brussels sprouts, all kinds of dried beans, onions, garlic, carrots, tomatoes, berries, grapes, fresh pineapple, nuts. I add onions and garlic to almost any dish that I make for dinner or lunch.

An analysis of my oatmeal breakfast; Everyone knows the benefits of old fashioned oatmeal, when I add dehydrated goji berries it adds protein and also a terrific antioxidant, goji is listed as a super food. I add Salba; it is a seed that is thought by some to be a perfect whole food. It is a rich source of omega 3 and fiber. Salba contains many of the vitamins and minerals you need each day. I love this seed. If you do not eat oatmeal, add this to your salad. Most everyone knows the advantage of adding nuts to any dish and also dried fruit, such as raisins. Coconut is another food that is an almost perfect food then honey, the 'fruit of the bee' adds to the taste and the benefits of this meal. Freshly ground flax seed is a great thing to add to oatmeal or to a salad, it provides you with the fat that aids your hormones and many other things, it is considered to be a good cancer fighter too. I grind my own in a coffee grinder because it can get old really fast after the seeds are ground. It can be kept in the freezer.

Anyone could have a good nutrition program by just eating this meal; it is so full of nutrition.

Things in my pantry:

- *Oils: olive oil, coconut oil, Mac nut oil, grape seed oil, walnut oil, unsalted butter (keep refrigerated) oils need to be in a cool dark place*
- *Apple cider vinegar*
- *Himalayan salt and sea salt*
- *Sweeteners: agava syrup, stevia, honey and molasses, a small container of raw sugar*
- *Spices: cumin, cinnamon, black pepper, cayenne pepper, oregano, basil , turmeric, ginger, dill, curry, rosemary, thyme*
- *Dried fruits: raisins, dried cranberries, dried pineapple, other dried fruits according to what I want at the time*
- *Nuts: walnuts, pecans, almonds, unsweetened coconut, cacao*

- *Old fashioned oatmeal, brown rice, assorted dried beans and peas, spinach pasta*
- *Assorted teas including neem tea and tulsi tea*
- *Canned goods including organic tomato sauces. Tomato products are always purchased in glass containers.*
- *Coffee beans*

My medicine cabinet:

- *Tea tree oil*
- *Vinegar*
- *Food grade hydrogen peroxide, many good uses including foot soaks*
- *Oil of oregano*
- *Olive leaf extract*
- *Zyflamend to take if I have inflammation*
- *Boric acid to use for foot soaks and cleanses*
- *Baking soda*
- *Aspirin*
- *Traumeel an anti inflammatory and pain supplement*
- *A supplement containing, glucosamine, condrontin MSM and hylauronic acid to use for joint discomfort*
- *Theratears eye drops and Similasan eye drops*
- *Neem leaves and oil*
- *Vicks Vaporub*

You will decide what you want in your medicine cabinet; I just wanted to share most of the things in mine.

"Folk Medicine": just wanted to share a few of the treatments I use frequently.

Foot soaks:

- *Hydrogen peroxide foot soak, Water 20 parts, Hydrogen Peroxide (food grade) 3% 1 part, one teaspoon Salt (Epsom salt or sea or table salt). Soak your feet for 20 minutes to relieve aching feet, improve circulation in feet, ankles and lower legs, for healing cracked skin, fungus or bacterial infections, or eliminate odor.*
- *If you do not have Hydrogen peroxide, use Hot Epsom Salt soaks.*

There are some resources that suggest using hot foot soaks for relieving most disease including the common cold.

- *Vicks Vaporub: all the years that I have lived, I am never without my Vicks, I use it in my nose to keep it from drying out and I rub it on my hands and feet at night. Even it is not a cure all, it makes me feel better. It is also an anti fungal so keeps toenails and fingernails free of fungus*

Sinus Cleanse:

- *Use warm salt water or a sinus cleanser to clean your nasal passages daily and especially when you have infections or sinus discomfort. It is easy to do as you shower.*

There are many more of these remedies but I just wanted to give you a few suggestions.

Chapter Eight

If I had trauma or illness

If I became ill here are a few things I would do to improve my chances of becoming well.

- *Do some research to find the correct supplements and food that would combat my illness. Example; diabetes, take oil of oregano, alpha lipoic acid, chromium picolinate, milk thistle, cinnamon, etc.*
- *I would seek out all the healing arts; Energy healing, Qigong, Acupuncture, Chiropractic, Hyperbaric oxygen, Eft, EWOT. Tai chi, Special meditations, NAET, Reflexology, Reiki, Yoga*
- *Change to a complete antifungal/anti inflammatory nutrition program*
- *Be certain to do all the cleanses and check for heavy metals, also do hormone testing*
- *Check on admittance to an alternative wellness center and if I could afford it I would go to a center such as; The Whitaker Wellness Center or one I have found in my research. If I had fibromyalgia or chronic fatigue, I would go to Dr. Tietelbaum's center, if a brain disorder; Dr. Perlmutter, etc.*
- *Get a massage and go for an infrared sauna*
- *I would search out a health care advocate to help find the right modalities for the illness.*

I am going to include some articles I have written on how to avoid osteoporosis, how to treat your pet, and other articles I have written.

Osteoporosis:

1. Get at least 30 minutes of sunshine daily. Don't let your love for sunscreen assist you in "giving" osteoporosis to your body

2. Eat fruits and vegetables that are colorful and don't overcook them, eat as near raw as possible
3. Avoid sodas, diet or otherwise and never smoke
4. Exercise daily using light weights
5. Avoid anti acids, they destroy the Hydrochloric acid in your stomach, thereby destroying the pathway for your calcium to reach you cells
6. Take supplements, including magnesium, boron and vitamin D. Magnesium does better as a spray or rub-on because then it goes directly to your cells.
7. Have your vitamin D and hormone levels read, if possible have your physician send you to a compounding pharmacist for the hormone levels, if you want you can order a vitamin D test on-line.
8. Be cautious about the amount and kind of supplemental calcium you take, it could end up as plaque in your arteries

Avoiding sprains, strains and fractures:

- Keep house free of clutter, rugs, etc.
- Never walk in the dark, turn lights on and use night lights
- Pick up your feet when you walk, don't shuffle you feet or drag them, lift with each step
- Clean up spills rapidly
- Train your pets not to walk or stand near your feet (this is very difficult)
- Observe the world around you, always be aware of your surroundings
- Use hand rails where available
- Keep your vision keen
- Wear shoes that are good for walking
- Good nutrition and exercise
- Keep your bones healthy with adequate sunshine, magnesium, boron, vitamin C, calcium and vitamin D
- Keep hormones at correct levels

Don't Be "Old"
There are 3 parts to getting "old", look old, act old and feel old

Don't Act old:

- Enjoy the small things in life: laugh and play a lot

- Use excellent posture, poor posture makes you feel old and act old
- Keep eyes bright
- If you have a hearing problem, wear a device to improve your hearing. So many people I know act old because they refuse to wear a device for hearing and anyone who cannot hear what is going on, acts old.
- Keep improving your brain and you will fit in everywhere you go and will not be considered old

Don't Look old:

- Keep skin well hydrated and take care of teeth and nails
- Never wear drab colors or poor fitting clothing
- Do not go on any rapid weight loss programs, people who have rapid weight loss look old, old, old

Don't Feel old:

- Eat well, take supplements, as we age we need more vitamins, minerals and herbs to stay healthy
- Observe your body for signs of disease/illness; color of urine (lemonade yellow), bowel movements (soft, well formed and at least one a day preferably more often), etc.
- Exercise to stay flexible and strong
- Do something great for others at least daily
- Be passionate about a hobby
- Go to spa, do relaxation exercises, deep breathing exercises and revive your brain
- Care for a pet
- Avoid accidents, if you have an injury, you will not only feel old but you will literally age in your whole body.
- Keep positive attitude
- If you have pain use a homeopathic pain killer, one is: traumeel
- There are some treatments adding oxygen to your exercise program called: EWOT

Avoid Infections:

- Wash hands frequently and keep them away from your face and hair if possible, I would suggest neem soap
- Eat lots of fresh fruits and vegetables, if you don't get enough green vegetable, take a green supplement

- Be certain that your supplements contain lots of antioxidants, fish oil and co enzyme Q10
- If you have been exposed to an illness, take oil of oregano and eat more garlic and onions
- Drink plenty of liquids
- Avoid sugar, bacteria and most diseases love sugar. Sweeten with Stevia or honey. Do not use the little "pink or blue packages", they are poison
- Get plenty of rest, fresh air and sunshine
- Have an air filtration system for your home and office
- Breathe deeply several times a day
- Wash nasal passages daily with a salt solution

Keeping your pets healthy and happy: I treat my pets as royal subjects who live in their castle (sometimes called my house) I only live here to keep them happy.

About 7 years ago I received a Yorkie puppy, I named Harry Potter. He was bought for me by my daughter-in-law and grandson. I had never had a pure bred dog and found that Harry was prone to lots of allergies. I did a lot of research to find what worked for him and I am going to write a list of things I do. I have since become rescue haven and have ended up with 14 dogs, many of them are pure breeds but families had to leave them because they could no longer keep them. I have pugs, doxies, poms, my yorkie and a couple of mixes. 3 cats have found me, a horse, a mini mule, a pygmy goat and a couple of chickens. They are all treated like royalty and I am their servant.

I do not give them any food except Life abundance made by a holistic vet at: www.healthypetnet.com/freddie and I keep them healthy not only for their happiness but to keep from paying vet bills.

Here are some of my suggestions (the way I do it):

- First thing every morning we take a trip to the back yard for evacuation and a bit of exercise, I have 3 doggy doors but they prefer to have a human with them when they are out doors.
- They come to the kitchen for their treat of the day which is a meat ball: ground meat, oatmeal, fish oil, eggs and if I have left over vegetables they are ground up and added. I freeze them in mini muffin tins and when I serve them, most of the dogs like the exercise of eating them frozen, some dogs like them thawed so I thaw usually 5 of them.
- Fresh water and food in their bowl (older dogs are fed softened food with some canned food added) then

- Back outside for some exercise while I feed the cats and the livestock.
- Cats are fed healthy pet net cat food both dry and wet, also given an antioxidant vitamin they love
- When the dogs come inside we listen to classical music while they each get combed for fleas and anything else that may have gotten into their fur and I check each for skin problems and check their ears.
- My ear wash for the dogs contain: alcohol, vinegar, oil of oregano and tea tree oil
- Vitamin supplements are given according to need, usually the poms are in need of a skin and coat preparation and the older dogs need the agility supplement. I also give my dogs eye drops to prevent cataracts
- There are weekly shampoos and neem oil is used for any skin conditions, nails are also trimmed. Don't have to trim the nails of the doxies very often because they love to dig, I have lots of holes in my yard and they love it.
- Dental care and digestive care is given about 1 time a week with raw bones cut at the butcher shop, it is a thigh bone cut into 1 inch slices and is frozen. They love chewing off all the meat, getting the bone marrow out and then the bone is left to chew on later just for fun and exercise.
- As you can imagine, floor quilts, pillows and dog beds are washed at least one time a week

My animals are important to me and I do everything I can to keep them happy and healthy.

Chapter Nine

How to check for wellness progress

Measuring your wellness:

Probably the dream would be to have a health care advocate, do your research, find your practitioner, put together your program and "feed it to you" as a complete program. This would be nice but I firmly believe you will enjoy it more if you have full participation in your wellness program.

You can measure your own wellness but I would suggest that you ask your health advocate to recommend the tests your health care provider needs to do to assist you in assessing your wellness. Here are a few suggestions on how to listen and find out how you are doing.

Skin, Hair, Nails: look at their appearance and how do they feel; skin pink and without blemish, hair shinny and no flaking, strong pink nails.

Skeletal system: Joints and muscles, - flexible with no pain, swelling or discomfort

Circulatory system; Blood flow, no chest discomfort, and no leg pain, etc.

Digestive system: no acid reflux, good digestion without excessive gas or discomfort when you eat, at least one large soft formed bowel movement a day, urinary system check: urine should be lemonade colored, no pain or urgency.

Respiratory system: sinus and lungs-easy deep breathing without pain, no stuffy or draining nasal passages and no cough. This is so important, heavy smokers sometimes almost smother to death and it is so painful to watch them suffer. I think of all the ones I watched in pain, every time I take a deep breath.

Ears, Eyes, and Head: No discomfort, good hearing and good vision-no dryness or redness of the eyes, etc.

I also want to encourage you to have good dental health, if you have lost a lot of teeth, you will not chew well and that keeps you from having the correct enzymes to digest your food well.

Sometimes I change my program because of what happened to someone else. My sister had a bad experience with cataract surgery so I determined not to ever have cataracts. I went to the web and found Dr. Kondrot and started using his protocol. I was especially interested because my little Yorkie, Harry Potter had a cataract that vets told me nothing could be done to prevent, I started him on Dr. Kondrot's protocol and he is doing well also.

As you assess each part of your body, listen to your body, it will tell you what needs to be changed to make you well.

My body "talks to me" and I listen because I will feel sluggish, have some muscle discomfort, have inflammation in my eye or will sometimes just feel, "down in the dumps". Then I must figure out where I messed up and change my daily program. Sometimes I just have to remember what I have been forgetting to do, such as; doing my exercises consistently, eating sugar or too much grain. I can usually figure it out without much difficulty. I always enjoy the fact that I am a "CSI", crime scene investigator; I am investigating the cause of my problems.

I feel that the most important thing you can do to stay well is to listen to your body. This old mema plans to listen and stay well.

Staying well is an ongoing battle but it is worth it. To find out why you need to have ultimate wellness, go visit a nursing home. Someone told me that their supplements were too expensive, consider the cost of a prescription drug and the side effects of a prescription drug and then decide if your supplements are too expensive. Quality of life is what we desire and there is no quality of life if you do not feel well every day. Listen to your body and be well!

Chapter Ten

Feedback

I warned you by the title, that this book was going to be my ramblings and I think you will agree, I ramble and do not organize very well. I do hope you learned something from my ramblings and enjoyed them.

I would love for you to share, your goals, your successes and your ideas with me:

www.freddiemema@hotmail.com I would hope that this little book will help fill your bucket and that in turn you will fill someone else's bucket.

I would also suggest that you take this book along with a little journal and give as a gift to someone who wants to <u>be well</u>.

Freddie Martin Arbuthnot: A retired registered nurse, graduated from Arkansas Baptist School of Nursing 1955, and attended University of the Ozarks and University of Arkansas, Little Rock, Arkansas: Studied natural healing and holistic health for the past 30 years. She has completed studies in many of the energy healing modalities and nutrition, and continues to study all aspects of natural healing. She considers herself to be a purveyor of wisdom, the vehicle for people to learn about wellness learned from the experts. She is a student open to learning for the remainder of her life.

Mother of 4 and grandmother of 2; has been a widow since 1982.

Medical positions: Hospital medical/surgical nurse, Intensive care nurse, Director of Nursing, Administrator of health care facility, nursing manager of rehabilitation hospital, Corporate health and wellness coordinator, summer camp nurse, home health nurse

Additional jobs: Operator of day care/nursery school, advocate for preschool education, Mary Kay Beauty consultant, Event planner, pampered chef, desk clerk and breakfast hostess for motel, Master bear builder for Build A Bear, workers' compensation claims manager, real estate sales person, photo lab tech, pet sitter/advocate for animal health,, employment counselor, sales clerk,

She has lived in Arkansas, Missouri, Colorado, and Texas.